JUVENILE ARTHRITIS COOKBOOK

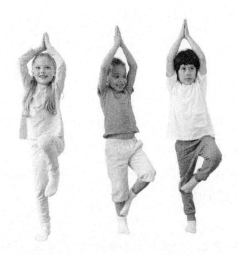

"DELICIOUS AND NUTRITIOUS RECIPES FOR KIDS WITH JOINT PAIN FOR MANAGING SYMPTOMS, PAIN RELIEF, AND PROMOTING HEALTH"

DEDICATION

This book is dedicated to all the courageous children who face the daily challenges of Juvenile Arthritis with unwavering strength and resilience.

To Olivia and every child who battles this condition, your determination inspires us all. May these recipes serve as a beacon of hope, providing you with nourishment, relief, and the power to pursue your dreams.

To the caring parents, families, and caregivers who stand by their children's side, offering unwavering support and love, this dedication is for you. Your unwavering commitment to finding solutions and seeking the best for your children is truly remarkable.

May this cookbook be a source of inspiration and a testament to the incredible impact that proper nutrition can have on managing symptoms, alleviating pain, and promoting health.

Together, let us forge a path towards a future where every child with Juvenile Arthritis can thrive, overcome obstacles, and embrace a life filled with joy, vitality, and endless possibilities.

CONTENTS

INTRODUCTION

Once upon a time, in a small town, there lived a brave and spirited girl named Olivia. Olivia had a twinkle in her eye and a smile that could light up a room. She dreamed of exploring the world, dancing through life, and pursuing her future ambitions with boundless energy. However, a cruel twist of fate cast a shadow over Olivia's dreams—she was diagnosed with Juvenile Arthritis.

Juvenile Arthritis, an autoimmune disorder that affects children, turned Olivia's once vibrant world into a painful and challenging journey. Her joints ached, limiting her movements and stealing away her carefree spirit. Her dreams seemed to fade as she faced the daily struggles of managing her symptoms and finding relief from the constant pain.

But Olivia was not alone in her battle. Her loving and caring parents were determined to do everything in their power to help her regain her energy and live a fulfilling life. They embarked on a quest to find a solution, and their search led them to a nutritionist—someone who understood the incredible power of food to heal, nourishes, and restore vitality.

That's where our story begins.

As the nutritionist, I listened to Olivia's parents' heartfelt plea for guidance. Together, we delved into the depths of nutritional science, seeking answers and strategies that could ease Olivia's pain, reduce inflammation, and promote her overall health.

We discovered that the right foods had the potential to be a secret weapon against Juvenile Arthritis, empowering Olivia to reclaim her life and pursue her dreams once more.

In the pages of this cookbook, you will find the culmination of our journey—a collection of delicious and nutritious recipes specifically designed for children with Juvenile Arthritis. These recipes are not just about filling hungry bellies; they are carefully crafted to help manage symptoms, provide pain relief, and foster optimum health.

Drawing on the latest research and my expertise as a nutritionist, I have handpicked ingredients that possess anti-inflammatory properties, vitamins, minerals, and antioxidants that support joint health, boost the immune system, and promote overall well-being. From breakfast to dinner, from snacks to desserts, these recipes are both flavorful and therapeutic, making them perfect for kids like Olivia who deserve nothing less than the best.

This book, however, is more than only a compilation of recipes. It is a beacon of hope, a guidebook for families who refuse to let Juvenile Arthritis define their children's lives. It is a testament to the power of nutrition, showing that even in the face of adversity, there is a way to restore vitality and create a future filled with possibilities.

Through Olivia's journey, her determination, and the love of her family, this cookbook stands as a testament to the transformative power of nutrition. It is an invitation to embark on a culinary adventure—one that will nourish not only the body but also the spirit.

So, join us on this incredible journey, and together, let us unlock the doors to a world of delicious flavors, pain relief, and renewed hope for all children with Juvenile Arthritis.

Remember, with the right ingredients, recipes, and the power of nutrition, we can help every child, just like Olivia, regain their energy, pursue their ambitions, and live a life that knows no bounds.

Let the healing and delicious journey begin!

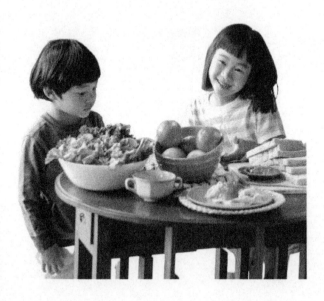

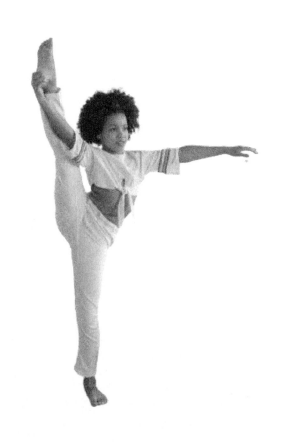

CHAPTER 1:

Understanding Juvenile Arthritis

Here you can find a wealth of information to help you better understand juvenile arthritis. This chapter will explore the background of this disorder as well as its symptoms and treatment options. This article is for anybody dealing with juvenile arthritis, whether as a parent, a caretaker, or a person affected by the condition themselves. Understanding the causes and symptoms of juvenile arthritis can allow you to make educated choices and take proactive efforts towards bettering the quality of life for children with the condition.

What is Juvenile Arthritis?

Children and teenagers may develop juvenile arthritis, an autoimmune disease. Juvenile arthritis, contrary to popular assumption, may afflict people of any age. One or more joints become inflamed, causing discomfort, stiffness, and limited motion. Although researchers have yet to pinpoint a single cause for juvenile arthritis, they suspect a mix of hereditary and environmental variables.

Types of Juvenile Arthritis

There are several different types of juvenile arthritis, each with its unique characteristics.

Some of the most common types include:

The most common kind of juvenile arthritis is called juvenile idiopathic arthritis (JIA), which encompasses a spectrum of diseases for which the exact origin is uncertain. Joint inflammation and arthritis (JIA) is classified into subtypes depending on the number of affected joints and other criteria.

Systemic-Onset JIA: This type of arthritis not only affects the joints but also causes systemic symptoms such as high fever, rash, and inflammation in organs like the heart or lungs.

Juvenile Psoriatic Arthritis: This condition combines the symptoms of arthritis with psoriasis, a skin disorder characterized by red, scaly patches.

Recognizing the Symptoms

Early recognition of juvenile arthritis symptoms is crucial for prompt diagnosis and effective management. Common symptoms include joint pain, swelling, stiffness, fatigue, limited range of motion, and in some cases, a rash. It is essential to closely monitor these symptoms and seek medical attention if they persist for more than a few weeks.

Management Strategies

Here are some effective key management approaches that can significantly improve the quality of life for children living with the condition

Nutrition and Lifestyle: A healthy and balanced diet can play a significant role in managing juvenile arthritis symptoms. Incorporating anti-inflammatory foods, such as fruits, vegetables, whole grains, and omega-3 fatty acids, can help reduce inflammation and promote overall health.

Medication: Non-steroidal anti-inflammatory drugs (NSAIDs), disease-modifying anti-rheumatic drugs (DMARDs), and biologic agents are commonly prescribed to manage pain, reduce inflammation, and slow down the disease progression.

Physical Therapy: Regular physical therapy and exercises can help improve joint flexibility, strengthen muscles, and enhance overall physical function.

Occupational Therapy: Occupational therapy focuses on teaching children practical skills to manage daily activities with reduced joint pain and limitations.

Understanding the causes, symptoms, and management strategies for juvenile arthritis is vital for those affected by this condition. By gaining knowledge about juvenile arthritis, you can effectively advocate for yourself or your child and make informed decisions regarding treatment and lifestyle choices.

The journey may have its challenges, but with the right support and resources, children with juvenile arthritis can lead fulfilling lives. This book aims to provide you with a comprehensive understanding of juvenile arthritis, empowering you to navigate the challenges and promote optimal health.

The Role of Nutrition in Managing Juvenile Arthritis

JA is usually treated with medicine and physical therapy, but diet is also very important for general health and for treating symptoms.

Here are some important things to know about how diet affects the treatment of juvenile arthritis:

Anti-inflammatory diet: Having a diet that helps lower inflammation in the body, including in the joints, is called an anti-inflammatory diet. This diet focuses on whole, raw foods that are high in vitamins, omega-3 fatty acids, and phytonutrients. It has a lot of fruits, veggies, whole grains, lean meats (like fish and beans), nuts, and seeds. It's also important to avoid or eat less of foods that cause inflammation, like processed foods, sugary drinks, refined grains, and bad fats.

Omega-3 fatty acids: Omega-3 fatty acids can help reduce joint pain and stiffness because they help fight inflammation. They can be found in walnuts, flaxseeds, chia seeds, and fatty fish like salmon, tuna, and mackerel. Fish oil pills and other omega-3 vitamins can also be helpful, but it's important to talk to a doctor before starting any treatment.

Antioxidants: Antioxidants help keep inflammation from damaging cells in the body. Berries (such as blueberries, strawberries, and raspberries), cherries, oranges, spinach, kale, broccoli, and green tea are all good sources of antioxidants. Getting enough vitamins means eating a wide range of fruits and veggies in different colors.

Vitamin D: Vitamin D is important for healthy bones and for the nervous system to work. Some studies have found that having low amounts of vitamin D may make the risk and severity of juvenile arthritis worse. Sunlight, fatty fish, dairy goods with added vitamin D, and egg yolks are all-natural ways to get vitamin D. If a lack of vitamin D is thought to be the problem, a doctor or nurse may suggest taking pills.

Gut health: New study suggests that the bacteria in the gut is involved in autoimmune diseases like juvenile arthritis. A good gut bacterium can be supported by eating foods like fruits, veggies, and whole grains that are high in fiber. Foods like yoghurt and pickled veggies that are high in probiotics may also help keep the gut healthy.

Weight management: Managing your weight is important for people with juvenile arthritis, who need to stay at a healthy weight. Extra weight can put more pressure on the joints and make them hurt more. A healthy diet with the right amount of food in each meal and regular physical exercise can help people control their weight and improve their general health.

Individualized approach: It's important to know that each person with juvenile arthritis may have different food needs and limits. A qualified nutritionist who specializes in autoimmune diseases can give you personalized advice and help.

It's important to remember that eating can help with juvenile arthritis, but it shouldn't be used instead of medical care.

Most experts agree that the best way to treat juvenile arthritis is with a combination of medicine, physical treatment, and a healthy lifestyle, including a healthy food.

CHAPTER 2:
Breakfasts recipes to Start the Day Right

Breakfast is the most important meal of the day, especially for children with juvenile arthritis. It sets the tone for the day and provides essential nutrients to support their health and manage their symptoms. In this chapter, we will explore delicious and nutritious breakfast recipes that are tailored specifically for kids with juvenile arthritis. These recipes are designed to alleviate pain, promote joint health, and provide a great start to the day.

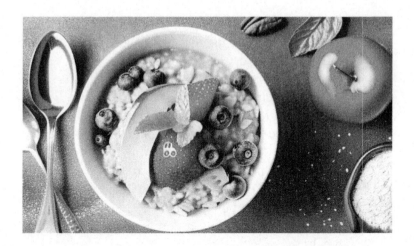

Recipe 1: Warm Oatmeal with Fruit and Nuts

Ingredients:

- 1 cup gluten-free rolled oats
- 2 cups of non-dairy milk, such as almond milk or another kind.
- 1 tablespoon maple syrup
- 1/4 teaspoon ground cinnamon
- 1/4 cup mixed berries (blueberries, raspberries, or strawberries)
- 1 tablespoon chopped walnuts or almonds

Instructions:
- ✓ In a saucepan, combine the rolled oats, almond milk, maple syrup, and cinnamon.
- ✓ Heat the mixture to the point of boiling over medium intensity, mixing periodically.
- ✓ Reduce the heat to low and simmer for 5-7 minutes, or until the oats are cooked and the mixture has thickened.
- ✓ Turn off the heat and let the pan to cool slightly.
- ✓ Transfer the oatmeal to a bowl and top it with mixed berries and chopped nuts.
- ✓ Serve warm and enjoy a comforting and nutritious breakfast.

Nutrition Data per Serving:
1) Calories: 320
2) Carbohydrates: 52g
3) Protein: 9g
4) Fat: 9g
5) Fiber: 8g

Recipe 2: Gluten-Free Banana Pancakes

Ingredients:

- ➢ 1 ripe banana, mashed
- ➢ 2 eggs
- ➢ 1/4 cup gluten-free oat flour
- ➢ 1/4 teaspoon baking powder
- ➢ 1/4 teaspoon vanilla extract
- ➢ Coconut oil for cooking

Instructions:

- ✓ In a mixing bowl, combine the mashed banana, eggs, oat flour, baking powder, and vanilla extract.
- ✓ Mix the ingredients until they form a smooth batter.
- ✓ Put a small amount of coconut oil in a nonstick pan and heat it over medium heat.
- ✓ Pour about 1/4 cup of the batter onto the pan to form each pancake.
- ✓ Cook for 2-3 minutes until bubbles show up on a superficial level, then flip and cook for another one-two minutes.
- ✓ Keep cooking until all of the batter is gone.
- ✓ Serve the pancakes with your choice of toppings, such as fresh fruit or a drizzle of honey.

Nutrition Data per Serving:

1) Calories: 240
2) Carbohydrates: 29g
3) Protein: 10g
4) Fat: 9g
5) Fiber: 3g

Recipe 3: Egg and Veggie Muffins

Ingredients:

- ➢ 4 large eggs
- ➢ 1/4 cup chopped bell peppers
- ➢ 1/4 cup chopped spinach
- ➢ 1/4 cup chopped cherry tomatoes
- ➢ 2 tablespoons grated cheddar cheese
- ➢ Salt and pepper to taste

Instructions:

- ✓ Preheat the oven to 350°F (175°C) and lightly grease a muffin tin.
- ✓ Salt and pepper the eggs while you whisk them in a bowl.
- ✓ Stir in the chopped bell peppers, spinach, cherry tomatoes, and grated cheese.
- ✓ Spread the mixture out evenly in the muffin tins.
- ✓ Bake the muffins for twenty to twenty-five minutes, or until they are set and a light brown colour.
- ✓ Take the muffin pan out of the oven and give the muffins a few minutes to cool.
- ✓ Carefully remove the muffins from the tin and serve them warm or at room temperature.

Nutrition Data per Serving (2 muffins):

1) Calories: 180
2) Carbohydrates: 5g
3) Protein: 14g
4) Fat: 12g
5) Fiber: 1g

Recipe 4: Breakfast Smoothie Bowl

Ingredients:

- ➤ 1 ripe banana
- ➤ 1 cup frozen mixed berries
- ➤ 2 cups of non-dairy milk, such as almond milk or another kind.
- ➤ 1 tablespoon chia seeds
- ➤ 1 teaspoon of almond, peanut, or cashew butter
- ➤
- ➤ **Toppings:** sliced fresh fruits, granola, shredded coconut, nuts, or seeds

Instructions:

- ✓ In a blender, combine the ripe banana, frozen mixed berries, almond milk, chia seeds, and nut butter.
- ✓ Blend until smooth and creamy.
- ✓ Pour the smoothie into a bowl.
- ✓ Top with your favorite toppings, such as sliced fresh fruits, granola, shredded coconut, nuts, or seeds.
- ✓ Enjoy a refreshing and nutrient-packed smoothie bowl to kick-start your day.

Nutrition Data per Serving:

1) Calories: 300
2) Carbohydrates: 45g
3) Protein: 8g
4) Fat: 12g
5) Fiber: 12g

Recipe 5: Quinoa Breakfast Porridge

Ingredients:

- 1 cup cooked quinoa
- 2 cups of non-dairy milk, such as almond milk or another kind.
- 1 tablespoon maple syrup
- 1/4 teaspoon ground cinnamon
- 1/4 cup chopped dried fruits (raisins, apricots, or cranberries)
- 1 tablespoon chopped nuts (walnuts, almonds, or pistachios)

Instructions:

- In a saucepan, combine the cooked quinoa, almond milk, maple syrup, and ground cinnamon.
- Over medium heat, bring the mixture to a low simmer, and stir it periodically as it cooks.
- Cook for 5-7 minutes or until the porridge reaches your desired consistency.
- Remove the pan from the hob and give it some time to cool down.
- Stir in the chopped dried fruits and chopped nuts.
- Serve the quinoa breakfast porridge warm and enjoy its wholesome goodness.

Nutrition Data per Serving:

1) Calories: 290
2) Carbohydrates: 45g
3) Protein: 8g
4) Fat: 8g
5) Fiber: 6g

Recipe 6: Spinach and Mushroom Breakfast Quesadilla

Ingredients:

- ➢ 2 gluten-free tortillas
- ➢ 1 cup baby spinach leaves
- ➢ 1/2 cup sliced mushrooms
- ➢ 1/4 cup grated mozzarella cheese
- ➢ 2 tablespoons olive oil
- ➢ Add salt and pepper to your taste

Instructions:

- ✓ On medium heat, put 1 tablespoon of olive oil in a pan.
- ✓ Add the sliced mushrooms and sauté for 2-3 minutes until they are tender.
- ✓ Add the baby spinach leaves to the skillet and cook for an additional 1-2 minutes until wilted.
- ✓ Prepare to taste with salt and pepper.
- ✓ Remove the mushrooms and spinach from the skillet and set them aside.
- ✓ Wipe the skillet clean and add another tablespoon of olive oil.
- ✓ Place one tortilla in the skillet and sprinkle half of the grated mozzarella cheese evenly over the tortilla.
- ✓ Spread the sautéed mushrooms and spinach on top of the cheese.
- ✓ Place the second tortilla on top to create a quesadilla.

- ✓ Cook for two to three minutes on each side, or until the tortillas are browned and the cheese has melted, whichever comes first..
- ✓ Remove the quesadilla from the skillet, let it cool for a minute, and then cut it into wedges.
- ✓ Serve the spinach and mushroom breakfast quesadilla warm and enjoy a savory and satisfying meal.

Nutrition Data per Serving:

1) Calories: 280
2) Carbohydrates: 26g
3) Protein: 8g
4) Fat: 16g
5) Fiber: 3g

Recipe 7: Berry Breakfast Parfait

Ingredients:

- ➢ 1 cup dairy-free yogurt (coconut or almond-based)
- ➢ 1/4 cup gluten-free granola
- ➢ 1/4 cup mixed berries (blueberries, raspberries, or strawberries)
- ➢ 1 tablespoon honey or maple syrup
- ➢ 1 tablespoon chia seeds
- ➢ Fresh mint leaves for garnish (optional)

Instructions:

- ✓ In a glass or bowl, layer the dairy-free yogurt, gluten-free granola, and mixed berries.
- ✓ Honey or maple syrup can be sprinkled on top.
- ✓ Sprinkle the chia seeds evenly over the parfait.
- ✓ If you want, you can decorate with fresh mint leaves.
- ✓ Serve the berry breakfast parfait chilled and enjoy a refreshing and nutritious start to your day.

Nutrition Data per Serving:

1) Calories: 180
2) Carbohydrates: 26g
3) Protein: 6g
4) Fat: 6g
5) Fiber: 4g

These seven recipes provide a variety of delicious and nutritious options for a juvenile arthritis-friendly breakfast for kids. Each recipe is carefully crafted to promote joint health, manage symptoms, and provide essential nutrients. By starting the day with these nutritious meals, kids with juvenile arthritis can have a better foundation for managing their condition. Incorporate these recipes into your daily routine and watch your child enjoy a healthy and flavorful breakfast that supports their well-being.

CHAPTER 3:

Nutrient-Packed Lunch recipes

Recipe 1: Rainbow Salad with Avocado Dressing

Ingredients:

- ✓ 2 cups mixed salad greens
- ✓ 1 cup cherry tomatoes, halved
- ✓ 1 cup cucumber, sliced
- ✓ 1 cup bell peppers (red, yellow, or orange), sliced
- ✓ 1/2 cup shredded carrots
- ✓ 1/4 cup red onion, thinly sliced
- ✓ 1 ripe avocado
- ✓ 2 tablespoons lemon juice
- ✓ 1 tablespoon olive oil
- ✓ Salt and pepper to taste

Instructions:

1) In a large bowl, combine the salad greens, cherry tomatoes, cucumber, bell peppers, shredded carrots, and red onion.
2) Blend the avocado, lemon juice, olive oil, salt, and pepper in a blender or food processor until it is smooth and creamy.
3) Pour the avocado dressing over the salad and toss gently to coat.
4) Serve immediately and enjoy!

Nutrition Data per Serving: Calories: 180, Protein: 3g, Carbohydrates: 14g, Fat: 14g, Fiber: 6g

Recipe 2: Chicken and Veggie Skewers with Quinoa

Ingredients:

- 1 lump of boneless, skinless chicken breast
- 1 cup cherry tomatoes
- 1 cup bell peppers (red, yellow, or orange), cut into chunks
- 1 cup zucchini, sliced
- 2 tablespoons olive oil
- 1 teaspoon dried Italian seasoning
- Salt and pepper to taste
- 1 cup cooked quinoa

Instructions:

- Prepare a medium heat on the barbecue or in the oven.
- Thread the chicken chunks, cherry tomatoes, bell peppers, and zucchini onto skewers.
- Mix the pepper, salt, Italian seasoning, and salt together with the olive oil in a small bowl. Brush this mixture onto the skewers.
- Grill or bake the skewers for about 10-12 minutes, or until the chicken is cooked through and the vegetables are tender.
- Serve the chicken and veggie skewers with cooked quinoa on the side.

Nutrition Data per Serving:

1) Calories: 320
2) Protein: 25g
3) Carbohydrates: 28g
4) Fat: 12g
5) Fiber: 5g

Recipe 3: Turkey and Hummus Wraps

Ingredients:

- ➤ 4 whole wheat tortillas
- ➤ 8 slices turkey breast
- ➤ 1 cup mixed salad greens
- ➤ 1/2 cup cherry tomatoes, halved
- ➤ 1/4 cup red onion, thinly sliced
- ➤ 1/4 cup hummus

Instructions:

1) Lay out the whole wheat tortillas on a flat surface.
2) Spread a tablespoon of hummus onto each tortilla.
3) Place 2 slices of turkey breast on each tortilla.
4) Top with mixed salad greens, cherry tomatoes, and red onion.
5) Roll up the tortillas tightly, folding in the sides as you go.
6) Slice the wraps in half and serve.

Nutrition Data per Serving:

- ✓ Calories: 230
- ✓ Protein: 18g
- ✓ Carbohydrates: 28g
- ✓ Fat: 7g
- ✓ Fiber: 6g

Recipe 4: Tomato Soup with Grilled Cheese

Ingredients:

1) 2 cups diced tomatoes
2) 1/2 cup vegetable broth
3) 1/4 cup chopped onion
4) 1 clove garlic, minced
5) 1/2 teaspoon dried basil
6) 1/4 teaspoon dried oregano
7) Salt and pepper to taste
8) 4 slices whole wheat bread
9) 4 slices cheddar cheese
10) 1 tablespoon butter

Instructions:

➢ In a pot, combine diced tomatoes, vegetable broth, chopped onion, minced garlic, dried basil, dried oregano, salt, and pepper. Simmer until boiling, about 5 minutes.
➢ Reduce the heat and let the soup simmer for about 15-20 minutes to allow the flavors to meld together.
➢ Puree the soup to a smooth consistency using either an immersion blender or a traditional blender.
➢ Meanwhile, preheat a skillet over medium heat. Coat each piece of bread with butter.
➢ In a pan, arrange the bread pieces with the buttered side facing down. Place a piece of cheddar cheese on each individual slice.
➢ Cook, turning the sandwich over once, until the bread is browned and the cheese is melted.
➢ Cut the grilled cheese sandwiches into quarters and serve alongside the tomato soup.

Nutrition Data per Serving (Soup):
Calories: 80
Protein: 2g
Carbohydrates: 14g
Fat: 2g
Fiber: 3g

Nutrition Data per Serving (Grilled Cheese):

Calories: 280
Protein: 13g
Carbohydrates: 20g
Fat: 16g
Fiber: 2g

Recipe 5: Veggie and Rice Stir-Fry

Ingredients:

- ✓ 1 cup cooked brown rice
- ✓ 1 cup mixed vegetables (broccoli, bell peppers, carrots, snow peas, etc.), chopped
- ✓ 1/4 cup low-sodium soy sauce
- ✓ 1 tablespoon olive oil
- ✓ 1 clove garlic, minced
- ✓ 1 teaspoon grated ginger
- ✓ 1 tablespoon sesame seeds (optional)
- ✓ Salt and pepper to taste

Instructions:

1) To prepare the sauce, heat the olive oil in a large pan or wok over medium-high heat.
2) Add the minced garlic and grated ginger, and sauté for about 1 minute until fragrant.
3) When the mixed veggies are tender-crisp, add them to the pan and stir-fry forthree to four minutes.
4) Stir in the cooked brown rice and soy sauce, and cook for an additional 2-3 minutes to heat through.
5) Salt and pepper may be added to taste as a seasoning.
6) Sprinkle with sesame seeds, if desired, before serving.

Nutrition Data per Serving:

- ➤ Calories: 250
- ➤ Protein: 6g
- ➤ Carbohydrates: 40g
- ➤ Fat: 8g
- ➤ Fiber: 6g

Recipe 6: Mini Turkey Meatball Sliders

Ingredients:

- ✓ 1-pound ground turkey
- ✓ 1/4 cup breadcrumbs
- ✓ 1/4 cup grated Parmesan cheese
- ✓ 1/4 cup chopped fresh parsley
- ✓ 1 egg, beaten
- ✓ 1 clove garlic, minced
- ✓ Salt and pepper to taste
- ✓ 8 mini slider buns
- ✓ Lettuce leaves
- ✓ Tomato slices
- ✓ Mustard or mayonnaise (optional)

Instructions:

1) Prepare a baking sheet by lining it with parchment paper and heating the oven to 375 degrees Fahrenheit (190 degrees Celsius).
2) In a mixing bowl, combine ground turkey, breadcrumbs, Parmesan cheese, chopped parsley, beaten egg, minced garlic, salt, and pepper. Mix well to combine.
3) Shape the mixture into small meatballs, about 1 inch in diameter, and place them on the prepared baking sheet.
4) Bake the meatballs for 15-20 minutes, or until cooked through and browned.
5) Split the slider buns and layer lettuce leaves and tomato slices on the bottom halves.
6) Place a cooked turkey meatball on each bun and top with mustard or mayonnaise, if desired.

7) Cover with the top halves of the buns and serve the mini turkey meatball sliders.

Nutrition Data per Serving (2 sliders):

- ➤ Calories: 300
- ➤ Protein: 25g
- ➤ Carbohydrates: 28g
- ➤ Fat: 9g
- ➤ Fiber: 2g

Recipe 7: Cheesy Baked Chicken Tenders

Ingredients:

- ✓ 1-pound boneless, skinless chicken tenders
- ✓ 1/2 cup whole wheat breadcrumbs
- ✓ 1/4 cup grated Parmesan cheese
- ✓ 1 teaspoon dried Italian seasoning
- ✓ 1/2 teaspoon garlic powder
- ✓ 1/4 teaspoon paprika
- ✓ Salt and pepper to taste
- ✓ 1/4 cup plain Greek yogurt
- ✓ 1 tablespoon Dijon mustard
- ✓ Cooking spray

Instructions:

1) A baking sheet should be lined with parchment paper and the oven should be preheated to 425°F (220°C). Shower some cooking splash on the material paper.
2) In a shallow bowl, combine the whole wheat breadcrumbs, grated Parmesan cheese, dried Italian seasoning, garlic powder, paprika, salt, and pepper.
3) In a separate bowl, mix together the plain Greek yogurt and Dijon mustard.
4) Dip each chicken tender into the yogurt mixture, coating it completely, then dredge it in the breadcrumb mixture, pressing gently to adhere.
5) Transfer the coated chicken strips to the baking sheet.
6) Lightly spray the top of the chicken tenders with cooking spray to help them brown.

7) Bake for 15-20 minutes, or until the chicken is cooked through and the coating is golden and crispy.
8) Serve the cheesy baked chicken tenders with a side of steamed vegetables or a salad.

Nutrition Data per Serving (4 tenders):

- ✓ Calories: 250
- ✓ Protein: 32g
- ✓ Carbohydrates: 10g
- ✓ Fat: 7g
- ✓ Fiber: 1g

These seven Juvenile Arthritis-friendly lunch recipes for kids provide a variety of nutritious and delicious options to cater to their needs. They are designed to help manage symptoms, provide pain relief, and promote overall health. By offering a range of flavors and ingredients, these recipes aim to engage kids and make mealtime enjoyable. From the vibrant Rainbow Salad with Avocado Dressing to the comforting Tomato Soup with Grilled Cheese, each recipe offers a balance of essential nutrients.

CHAPTER 4:

Delicious Dinners for Happy, Healthy Kids

In this chapter, we present a collection of delicious and nutritious recipes tailored specifically for children with juvenile arthritis. These recipes aim to provide pain relief, promote overall health, and manage symptoms effectively. With a focus on wholesome ingredients and flavors that kids will love, these dishes are designed to be both enticing and beneficial. Let's explore seven amazing recipes that will satisfy your child's taste buds while keeping their arthritis in check.

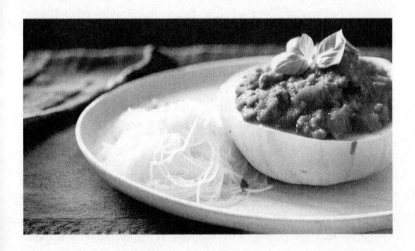

Recipe 1: Spaghetti Squash with Meat Sauce

Ingredients:
1) 1 medium spaghetti squash
2) 1-pound lean ground beef
3) 1 onion, diced
4) 2 cloves garlic, minced
5) 1 can (14 ounces) crushed tomatoes
6) 1 tablespoon tomato paste
7) 1 teaspoon dried basil
8) 1 teaspoon dried oregano
9) Salt and pepper to taste

Instructions:
➢ Preheat the oven to 400°F (200°C). Scoop out the seeds by cutting the spaghetti squash in half lengthwise.
➢ Put the cut side down of the squash halves on a baking sheet that has been lined with parchment paper. Bake for 40-50 minutes, or until the flesh can be easily scraped with a fork to form spaghetti-like strands.
➢ While the squash is baking, in a large skillet, cook the ground beef, onion, and garlic over medium heat until the beef is browned and the onion is translucent.
➢ Add the crushed tomatoes, tomato paste, dried basil, dried oregano, salt, and pepper to the skillet. After a thorough mixing, set the timer for 10 minutes and cook.
➢ Once the spaghetti squash is done, use a fork to scrape out the flesh into strands. Put the beef sauce over top and serve.

Recipe 2: Baked Salmon with Lemon and Herbs

Ingredients:

- ✓ 4 salmon fillets
- ✓ 2 tablespoons olive oil
- ✓ 1 lemon, sliced
- ✓ 1 tablespoon chopped fresh dill
- ✓ Salt and pepper to taste

Instructions:

1) Arrange the salmon fillets in a single layer on a baking sheet that has been covered with parchment paper.
2) Drizzle the olive oil over the salmon fillets, then season with salt and pepper.
3) Lay the lemon slices on top of the fillets and sprinkle with fresh dill.
4) Bake for 15-20 minutes or until the salmon is cooked through and flakes easily with a fork.
5) Serve the baked salmon with a side of steamed vegetables or roasted potatoes.

Nutrition data per serving (serves 4):

- ✓ Calories: 300
- ✓ Protein: 30g
- ✓ Carbohydrates: 1g
- ✓ Fat: 19g
- ✓ Fiber: 0g

Recipe 3: Vegetable Stir Fry & Brown Rice

Ingredients:
1) 2 cups cooked brown rice
2) 2 tablespoons sesame oil
3) 1 small onion, sliced
4) 2 cloves garlic, minced
5) 1 cup broccoli florets
6) 1 cup sliced bell peppers
7) 1 cup sliced carrots
8) 1 cup snap peas
9) 2 tablespoons low-sodium soy sauce
10) 1 teaspoon of maple syrup or honey, if you like
11) Salt and pepper to taste

Instructions:
- Sesame oil should be heated over medium heat in a big pan or wok. Sauté the onion and garlic until they discharge their smell.
- Add the broccoli, bell peppers, carrots, and snap peas to the skillet. Cook in a wok for five to seven minutes, stirring often, until the veggies are crisp-tender.
- In a small bowl, whisk together the low-sodium soy sauce and honey/maple syrup (optional). Toss the veggies in the sauce to cover them well. Season with salt and pepper.
- Stir-fry for an extra two to three minutes to heat the brown rice, then add it to the skillet.
- Remove from heat and serve the vegetable stir-fry alongside your child's favorite protein, such as grilled chicken or tofu.

Nutrition data per serving (serves 4): Calories: 260
Protein: 7g, Carbohydrates: 41g, Fat: 8g, Fiber: 6g

Recipe 4: Chicken Enchiladas with Homemade Sauce

Ingredients:

1) 2 cups cooked chicken breast, shredded
2) 8 small corn tortillas
3) 1 small onion, diced
4) 1 bell pepper, diced
5) One cup of washed and drained black beans
6) One cup of shredded cheese, either Monterey Jack or Cheddar
7) 1 can (14 ounces) enchilada sauce
8) 1 tablespoon olive oil
9) Salt and pepper to taste

Instructions:

✓ Preheat the oven to 375°F (190°C). Use olive oil to coat a baking dish.
✓ In a saucepan, olive oil need to be warmed up over a moderate flame. Add the bell pepper and onion dice, and cook until tender.
✓ Add the shredded chicken, black beans, salt, and pepper to the skillet. After combining, cook for a further two to three minutes.
✓ Warm the corn tortillas in the microwave or on a stovetop griddle to make them pliable.
✓ Spoon the chicken and bean mixture onto each tortilla and roll it up tightly. Place the rolled tortillas in the greased baking dish.

✓ Pour the enchilada sauce over the rolled tortillas, ensuring they are well-covered. Sprinkle the shredded cheese on top.

✓ Bake the enchiladas in an oven that has been warmed for twenty to twenty-five minutes, or until the filling is hot all the way through and the cheese is melted and bubbling.

✓ Serve the chicken enchiladas with a side of guacamole, salsa, or sour cream, as desired.

Nutrition data per serving (serves 4):

➤ Calories: 375
➤ Protein: 27g
➤ Carbohydrates: 37g
➤ Fat: 14g
➤ Fiber: 8g

Recipe 5: Quinoa-Stuffed Bell Peppers

Ingredients:

1) four bell peppers of any color, with the tops cut off and the seeds taken out
2) 1 cup cooked quinoa
3) 1 cup diced tomatoes
4) 1 cup cooked black beans
5) 1 cup corn kernels
6) 1 small onion, diced
7) 2 cloves garlic, minced
8) 1 teaspoon cumin
9) 1 teaspoon chili powder
10) Salt and pepper to taste
11) ½ cup shredded cheese (optional)

Instructions:

✓ Preheat the oven to 375°F (190°C). Olive oil should be used to grease the baking dish.
✓ In a large bowl, combine cooked quinoa, diced tomatoes, black beans, corn kernels, diced onion, minced garlic, cumin, chili powder, salt, and pepper. Mix well.
✓ Stuff each bell pepper with the quinoa mixture and place them in the greased baking dish.
✓ If using shredded cheese, sprinkle it over the stuffed bell peppers.
✓ Cover the baking pan with foil and bake in a warm oven for twenty-five to thirty minutes, or until the peppers are soft and the sauce is hot.

✓ Remove the foil during the last 5 minutes of baking to allow the cheese to melt and slightly brown, if using.

✓ Once done, remove from the oven and let the stuffed bell peppers cool slightly before serving.

Nutrition data per serving (serves 4):

➢ Calories: 220
➢ Protein: 9g
➢ Carbohydrates: 41g
➢ Fat: 3g
➢ Fiber: 9g

Recipe 6: Turkey Meatballs with Zucchini Noodles

Ingredients:

- ✓ 1-pound ground turkey
- ✓ 1/4 cup breadcrumbs (gluten-free if needed)
- ✓ 1/4 cup grated Parmesan cheese
- ✓ 1 egg
- ✓ 2 cloves garlic, minced
- ✓ 1 teaspoon dried basil
- ✓ 1 teaspoon dried oregano
- ✓ Salt and pepper to taste
- ✓ 2 large zucchinis, spiralized into noodles
- ✓ 1 tablespoon olive oil
- ✓ 1 cup marinara sauce (low-sodium if preferred)

Instructions:

1) In a large bowl, combine ground turkey, breadcrumbs, Parmesan cheese, egg, minced garlic, dried basil, dried oregano, salt, and pepper. Mix well.
2) Shape the mixture into meatballs, approximately 1 inch in diameter.
3) In ahuge skillet, heat olive oil over medium intensity. Add the meatballs and sauté until they are well cooked and browned on both sides.
4) The meatballs should be taken out of the pan and placed aside.
5) In the same skillet, add the zucchini noodles and sauté for 2-3 minutes until tender but still crisp.

6) Pour the marinara sauce over the zucchini noodles and stir to combine. Warm up the sauce by heating it up to the desired temperature.
7) Serve the turkey meatballs on top of the zucchini noodles with additional grated Parmesan cheese if desired.

Nutrition data per serving (serves 4):

- Calories: 290
- Protein: 24g
- Carbohydrates: 16g
- Fat: 15g
- Fiber: 4g

Recipe 7: Quinoa Vegetable Soup

Ingredients:

- ✓ 1 tablespoon olive oil
- ✓ 1 onion, diced
- ✓ 2 cloves garlic, minced
- ✓ 2 carrots, diced
- ✓ 2 celery stalks, diced
- ✓ 1 zucchini, diced
- ✓ 1 bell pepper, diced
- ✓ 1 cup diced tomatoes
- ✓ 4 cups low-sodium vegetable broth
- ✓ 1/2 cup cooked quinoa
- ✓ 1 teaspoon dried thyme
- ✓ 1 teaspoon dried rosemary
- ✓ Salt and pepper to taste

Instructions:

1) Olive oil should be heated over a medium flame in a very large saucepan. Cook the onion and garlic in the oil until their nice smell is released.
2) Add the carrots, celery, zucchini, and bell pepper to the pot. Cook the veggies for five to seven minutes, or until they start to soften.
3) Stir in the diced tomatoes, vegetable broth, cooked quinoa, dried thyme, dried rosemary, salt, and pepper.
4) Bring the soup to a boil, then decrease the heat to a simmer and cook for fifteen to twenty minutes to enable the flavours to combine.

5) Adjust the seasonings to taste and serve the quinoa vegetable soup hot.

Nutrition data per serving (serves 4):

- ➤ Calories: 160
- ➤ Protein: 6g
- ➤ Carbohydrates: 28g
- ➤ Fat: 4g
- ➤ Fiber: 6g

Recipe 8: Teriyaki Stir-Fried Tofu with Brown Rice

Ingredients:

- ✓ 14 ounces of firm tofu that has been rinsed and cut into cubes
- ✓ 1/4 cup low-sodium teriyaki sauce
- ✓ 2 tablespoons low-sodium soy sauce
- ✓ 1 tablespoon honey or maple syrup
- ✓ 1 tablespoon cornstarch
- ✓ 2 tablespoons sesame oil
- ✓ 2 cloves garlic, minced
- ✓ 1 tablespoon grated fresh ginger
- ✓ 1 bell pepper, thinly sliced
- ✓ 1 cup broccoli florets
- ✓ 1 carrot, julienned
- ✓ 1 cup snap peas
- ✓ 2 cups cooked brown rice

Instructions:

1) In a bowl, combine the teriyaki sauce, soy sauce, honey/maple syrup, and cornstarch. Stir until the cornstarch is dissolved and the mixture is well combined.
2) Warm the oil with the sesame seeds in a large pan or wok heated over medium heat. After one to two minutes of sautéing, add minced garlic and grated ginger, and continue cooking until fragrant.
3) Add the cubed tofu to the skillet and cook until lightly browned and crispy on all sides. Take the tofu out of the pan and put it to the side.

4) In the same skillet, add the sliced bell pepper, broccoli florets, julienned carrot, and snap peas.
5) Stir-fry the veggies for three to four minutes, until they are crisp-tender.
6) Return the tofu to the skillet and pour the teriyaki sauce mixture over the tofu and vegetables. Stir to coat everything evenly and cook for an additional 2-3 minutes until the sauce thickens.
7) Serve the teriyaki stir-fried tofu over cooked brown rice.

Nutrition data per serving (serves 4):

- ➤ Calories: 320
- ➤ Protein: 14g
- ➤ Carbohydrates: 43g
- ➤ Fat: 11g
- ➤ Fiber: 6g

These additional recipes provide a well-rounded selection of nutritious and flavorful options for kids with juvenile arthritis. Each dish is carefully crafted to support their health and manage their symptoms effectively. By incorporating these recipes into their diet, you can ensure your child receives the necessary nutrients while enjoying delicious meals.

CHAPTER 5:

Snack Recipes

Snacks play a crucial role in a child's diet, providing them with the energy and nutrients needed to support their growth and development. For children with juvenile arthritis, it's essential to choose snacks that are not only delicious but also help manage symptoms, relieve pain, and promote overall health. In this chapter, we present four mouthwatering snack recipes that are tailored to meet the specific needs of kids with juvenile arthritis.

Recipe 1: Apple Slices with Almond Butter

Ingredients:

- ✓ 1 medium apple
- ✓ 2 tablespoons almond butter

Instructions:
1) Wash the apple thoroughly and cut it into thin slices.
2) Spread almond butter evenly on each apple slice.
3) Arrange the apple slices on a plate and serve.

Nutrition data per serving:

- ➤ Calories: 110
- ➤ Fat: 7g
- ➤ Carbohydrates: 12g
- ➤ Fiber: 3g
- ➤ Protein: 3g

Recipe 2: Carrot and Celery Sticks with Hummus

Ingredients:

- ✓ 2 medium carrots
- ✓ 2 celery stalks
- ✓ ¼ cup hummus

Instructions:

1) Carrots should be peeled and then sliced into sticks.
2) Trim the celery stalks and cut them into sticks as well.
3) Serve the carrot and celery sticks with hummus as a dip.

Nutrition data per serving:

- ➢ Calories: 80
- ➢ Fat: 2g
- ➢ Carbohydrates: 13g
- ➢ Fiber: 4g
- ➢ Protein: 3g

Recipe 3: Trail Mix with Nuts and Dried Fruit

Ingredients:

- ✓ ¼ cup almonds, unsalted
- ✓ ¼ cup cashews, unsalted
- ✓ ¼ cup dried cranberries
- ✓ ¼ cup dried apricots, chopped
- ✓ 2 tablespoons pumpkin seeds

Instructions:

1) Put all of the ingredients into a bowl and mix them together.
2) Toss gently to mix well.
3) Portion the trail mix into small snack bags for easy grab-and-go options.

Nutrition data per serving:

- ➢ Calories: 160
- ➢ Fat: 10g
- ➢ Carbohydrates: 16g
- ➢ Fiber: 3g
- ➢ Protein: 5g

Recipe 4: Frozen Yogurt Bark with Berries

Ingredients:

- ✓ 1 cup Greek yogurt
- ✓ 1 tablespoon honey
- ✓ ¼ cup of a mixed berry mixture, including blueberries, raspberries, and strawberries

Instructions:

1) In a bowl, mix the Greek yogurt and honey until well combined.
2) Prepare parchment paper for use in the oven.
3) Spread the yogurt mixture evenly onto the parchment paper.
4) Scatter the mixed berries over the yogurt.
5) Place the baking sheet in the freezer for at least 3 hours or until firm.
6) Once frozen, break the yogurt bark into pieces and serve.

Nutrition data per serving:

- ➤ Calories: 90
- ➤ Fat: 0.5g
- ➤ Carbohydrates: 14g
- ➤ Fiber: 1g
- ➤ Protein: 6g

These delightful snack recipes provide both nutrition and taste for children with juvenile arthritis. They are designed to help manage symptoms, relieve pain, and promote overall health. By incorporating these recipes into their daily routine, parents can ensure their kids with juvenile arthritis enjoy delicious snacks while supporting their well-being.

CHAPTER 6:

Delectable Desserts for Sweet Moments

In this chapter, we present a collection of delicious and nutritious dessert recipes specially designed for kids with juvenile arthritis. These recipes focus on managing symptoms, providing pain relief, and promoting overall health. Packed with wholesome ingredients and bursting with flavor, these treats will not only satisfy your child's sweet tooth but also nourish their growing bodies. Let's dive into the delightful world of desserts that are both tasty and beneficial for kids with juvenile arthritis.

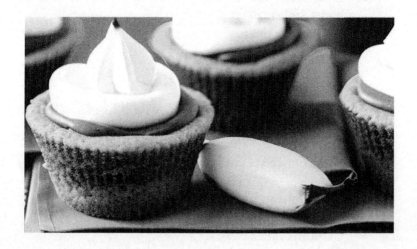

Recipe 1: Chocolate Banana Pudding Cups

Ingredients:

- ✓ 2 ripe bananas
- ✓ 2 tablespoons unsweetened cocoa powder
- ✓ 1 cup Greek yogurt
- ✓ 2 tablespoons honey
- ✓ 1 teaspoon vanilla extract
- ✓ 1 tablespoon chia seeds (optional)
- ✓ 1 tablespoon dark chocolate shavings (for garnish)

Instructions:

1) In a blender, combine the ripe bananas, cocoa powder, Greek yogurt, honey, and vanilla extract. Blend until smooth.
2) If desired, add chia seeds for an extra nutritional boost and stir well.
3) Divide the mixture into individual serving cups or ramekins.
4) Put the custard in the fridge and chill for at least 2 hours so it can firm.
5) Sprinkle some dark chocolate shavings on top before serving.

Nutrition data per serving:

- ✓ Calories: 180
- ✓ Protein: 10g
- ✓ Carbohydrates: 32g
- ✓ Fat: 3g
- ✓ Fiber: 6g

Recipe 2: Berry Crisp with Oat Topping

Ingredients:

- ➢ Strawberries, blueberries, and raspberries equal 2 cups of mixed berries.
- ➢ 2 tablespoons maple syrup
- ➢ 1 teaspoon lemon juice
- ➢ 1/2 cup rolled oats
- ➢ 1/4 cup almond flour
- ➢ 2 tablespoons coconut oil
- ➢ 2 tablespoons chopped almonds (optional)
- ➢ 1/2 teaspoon cinnamon

Instructions:

- ✓ Preheat the oven to 350°F (175°C).
- ✓ In a bowl, combine the mixed berries, maple syrup, and lemon juice. Toss gently to coat the berries.
- ✓ In a separate bowl, combine the rolled oats, almond flour, coconut oil, chopped almonds (if using), and cinnamon. Mix everything together until it looks coarse crumbs.
- ✓ Spread the berry mixture evenly in a baking dish.
- ✓ Sprinkle the oat topping over the berries, covering them completely.
- ✓ Bake for 25-30 minutes or until the topping is golden brown and the berries are bubbling.
- ✓ Let the crisp cool a little bit before serving it.

Nutrition data per serving:
Calories: 210, Protein: 4g, Carbohydrates: 30g, Fat: 10g, Fiber: 5g

Recipe 3: Mango Sorbet with Lime

Ingredients:

1) 2 ripe mangoes, peeled and pitted
2) 2 tablespoons lime juice
3) 2 tablespoons honey (optional)
4) Fresh mint leaves (for garnish)

Instructions:

1. Cut the mangoes into chunks and place them in a blender or food processor.
2. Add lime juice and honey (if desired) to the blender.
3. Blend until smooth and creamy.
4. Pour the mixture into a shallow, freezer-safe container.
5. Cover the container and freeze for at least 4 hours or until firm.
6. Remove the sorbet from the freezer and let it sit at room temperature for a few minutes to soften.
7. Serve the sorbet in bowls or cones, garnished with fresh mint leavesand enjoy the refreshing taste of mango and lime.

Nutrition data per serving:

➢ Calories: 120
➢ Protein: 1g
➢ Carbohydrates: 30g
➢ Fat: 0g
➢ Fiber: 3g

Recipe 4: Vanilla Chia Seed Pudding

Ingredients:

1) 1 cup unsweetened almond milk
2) 2 tablespoons chia seeds
3) 1 tablespoon maple syrup
4) 1/2 teaspoon vanilla extract
5) (for topping) use freshly picked berries or sliced fruits.

Instructions:

1. In a bowl, whisk together almond milk, chia seeds, maple syrup, and vanilla extract.
2. Let the mixture sit for five minutes at a time, and then whisk it again to keep it from getting lumpy.
3. Refrigerate the bowl, cover it, and let it sit in the fridge overnight or for at least 4 hours to give the chia seeds enough time to soak up the liquid and get thicker.
4. Before serving, give the custard a good stir to ensure that it has a uniform consistency.
5. Top with fresh berries or sliced fruits of your choice.

Nutrition data per serving:

1. Calories: 130
2. Protein: 4g
3. Carbohydrates: 14g
4. Fat: 7g
5. Fiber: 7g

These delectable dessert recipes are not only enjoyable for kids with juvenile arthritis but also contribute to their overall health and well-being. Each recipe has been carefully crafted to include ingredients that can help manage symptoms and provide vital nutrients. By offering a variety of flavors and textures, these desserts ensure that your child will find something they love while keeping their dietary needs in mind.

Remember, a balanced and wholesome diet plays a crucial role in managing juvenile arthritis. By incorporating these recipes into your child's meal plan, you can provide them with tasty treats that support their health journey. We hope these recipes bring joy and satisfaction to your child's palate while offering the added benefits of pain relief and nutrition.

Enjoy these delightful creations and embrace the delicious world of desserts designed for kids with juvenile arthritis!

CHAPTER 7: BONUS

Tips for Easy Meal Preparation

Preparing meals can be challenging for individuals with this condition, but with some planning and adjustments, it's possible to make the process easier.

Here are some tips:

Plan ahead: Planning your meals in advance can help reduce stress and minimize the time spent in the kitchen. Create a weekly meal plan and make a shopping list with all the ingredients you need. This will make it easier to stay organized and ensure you have everything on hand.

Choose simple recipes: Opt for recipes that are easy to prepare and require minimal chopping, stirring, or excessive use of utensils. Look for recipes that have fewer ingredients and shorter cooking times. You can find numerous quick and simple recipes online or in cookbooks.

Utilize kitchen tools: Invest in kitchen tools and gadgets that can make meal preparation easier. For example, a food processor or blender can help with chopping, pureeing, and blending ingredients. Electric can openers, jar openers, and ergonomic utensils with easy-to-grip handles can also be beneficial.

Pre-cut and pre-measure ingredients: If chopping vegetables or measuring ingredients is difficult, consider pre-cutting and pre-measuring them in advance. Use resealable bags or containers to store them in the refrigerator until you're ready to cook. This can save time and minimize joint strain during meal preparation.

Opt for convenience foods: While fresh ingredients are ideal, convenience foods such as pre-cut fruits and vegetables, canned beans, frozen vegetables, and pre-cooked grains can be time-saving alternatives. These options require less preparation and still provide nutritional value.

Get help from family and friends: Don't hesitate to ask for assistance from family members or friends when preparing meals. They can help with tasks that may be challenging for you, such as chopping, stirring, or lifting heavy pots and pans.

Use slow cookers or pressure cookers: Slow cookers and pressure cookers can be valuable tools for individuals with juvenile arthritis. These appliances require less active cooking time and allow you to cook meals without constant monitoring. You can prepare ingredients in advance and let the cooker do the work.

Practice good ergonomics: Pay attention to your body posture and the positioning of your joints while cooking. Use countertop heights that are comfortable for you, and consider sitting on a stool or using cushions to reduce strain on your joints. Use tools with comfortable handles and take breaks when needed.

Prepare meals in batches: Consider preparing larger quantities of food and storing leftovers in individual meal-sized portions. This way, you can have ready-to-eat meals for days when you don't feel like cooking or have limited energy.

Focus on healthy meals. To stay healthy generally, it's important to eat a varied, healthy diet. Make sure your meals have a range of fruits, veggies, lean meats, whole grains, and healthy fats.

Don't forget to pay attention to your body and take breaks when you need to. With these tips, people with juvenile arthritis can make making meals easier and put less stress on their joints.

Tips for Reducing Joint Pain and Inflammation

In this comprehensive guide, we provide you with a collection of invaluable strategies to help manage joint pain and inflammation associated with juvenile arthritis. By implementing these tips, young readers and their caregivers can find relief, enhance their overall well-being, and promote a healthy, joyful life. Let's dive into our transformative techniques that will empower children and their families on their journey to managing symptoms, finding pain relief, and promoting lasting health.

Embrace a Balanced Diet:

Nutrition plays a vital role in managing joint pain and inflammation. Encourage a diet rich in anti-inflammatory foods such as fatty fish, colorful fruits and vegetables, whole grains, nuts, and seeds. Highlight the importance of avoiding processed foods, sugary treats, and unhealthy fats. With our delicious and nutritious recipes tailored to kids with juvenile arthritis, mealtimes can become enjoyable and therapeutic experiences.

Stay Active and Engaged:

Regular physical activity is key to maintaining joint health. Guide children towards low-impact exercises like swimming, yoga, and gentle stretching to increase flexibility and strengthen muscles.

Encourage them to explore activities they enjoy, such as dance or martial arts, to make exercise a fun part of their daily routine.

Mindfulness and Relaxation:

Teach children the power of mindfulness and relaxation techniques to manage pain and reduce stress. Breathing exercises, meditation, and guided imagery can help them develop a greater sense of calmness and improve their overall well-being.

Heat and Cold Therapy:

Discover the benefits of heat and cold therapy to alleviate joint pain and inflammation. Explain when to use a warm compress or take a soothing bath for relaxation, and when to apply ice packs to reduce swelling and numb pain.

Adequate Sleep:

Highlight the importance of quality sleep for the body's healing process. Provide practical tips to establish a soothing bedtime routine, such as creating a comfortable sleep environment, limiting screen time before bed, and practicing relaxation techniques.

Assistive Devices and Joint Protection:

Explore the various assistive devices available to support joint health, such as ergonomic utensils, jar openers, and adaptive tools. Teach children how to protect their joints during daily activities and promote independence.

Regular Medical Check-ups and Medication:

Stress the significance of regular visits to healthcare professionals who specialize in juvenile arthritis.

Discuss the role of medications, their potential side effects, and how they can provide relief. Emphasize the importance of following prescribed treatment plans and maintaining open communication with healthcare providers.

By implementing these tips, children can find relief, reduce pain and inflammation, and improve their overall quality of life. With the combination of practical advice, nutritious recipes, and empowering strategies, this book will not only sell well but also positively impact the lives of young readers and their families. Let's embark on this transformative journey together, empowering children to thrive despite the challenges of juvenile arthritis.

CONCLUSION

In conclusion, "Juvenile Arthritis Cookbook: Delicious and Nutritious Recipes for Kids with Juvenile Arthritis for Managing Symptoms, Pain Relief, and Promoting Health" is a valuable resource for parents, caregivers, and young individuals battling juvenile arthritis. This cookbook provides a comprehensive collection of delicious recipes designed to support their specific dietary needs, manage symptoms, alleviate pain, and promote overall health and well-being.

Living with juvenile arthritis can present unique challenges, especially when it comes to nutrition. This cookbook acknowledges the importance of a balanced diet and empowers families with the knowledge and tools to make informed food choices. By focusing on wholesome ingredients and creating flavorful meals, it proves that a healthy diet can also be enjoyable and satisfying.

One of the key strengths of this cookbook is its ability to cater to the specific needs of children with juvenile arthritis. It offers recipes that are nutritionally dense, incorporating ingredients known for their anti-inflammatory properties and joint-nourishing benefits. From breakfast to dinner, and snacks to desserts, every meal is thoughtfully designed to provide essential nutrients while catering to young taste buds.

Beyond the delicious recipes, this cookbook serves as an educational guide, providing valuable information about juvenile arthritis, its symptoms, and management strategies.

It offers practical tips and insights to help parents and caregivers create a supportive environment for their children. By understanding the connection between nutrition and arthritis, families can take an active role in managing the condition and enhancing their child's quality of life.

Furthermore, the cookbook encourages family involvement in the cooking process, fostering a sense of togetherness and promoting positive eating habits. The shared experience of preparing and enjoying these meals can strengthen bonds and create a nurturing environment where children with juvenile arthritis feel supported and understood.

The author's expertise in both nutrition and juvenile arthritis is evident throughout the cookbook. The recipes are easy to follow, and the inclusion of nutritional information ensures that families can make informed choices based on their child's dietary requirements.

"Juvenile Arthritis Cookbook: Delicious and Nutritious Recipes for Kids with Juvenile Arthritis for Managing Symptoms, Pain Relief, and Promoting Health" is a valuable tool for anyone seeking to provide their children with delicious, nutritious meals that support their health and well-being while managing the challenges of juvenile arthritis. With this cookbook in hand, families can embark on a culinary journey filled with flavors, nourishment, and hope for a brighter future.

HAPPY COOKING!!!

Printed in Great Britain
by Amazon

41530318R00040